CRAFTY WITCH'S LITTLE BOOK OF APHRODISIACS

A QUICK LOOK INTO THE FOODS

OF LOVE

Hubble bubble,
Toil and trouble,
Read my little book,
And your sex drive will double

Since the beginning of time, humans, desiring to reach new heights of sexual

pleasure, have sought out aphrodisiac substances to foster intimacy, increase sexual desire, inspire fidelity, to enhance passion, promote endurance, and to increase fertility or virility.

I've chosen not to include much in the way of oysters. While they may be the first thing people think of when talking about aphrodisiacs, I just find that the least sexy thing on the planet is a shell full of salty, living snot!

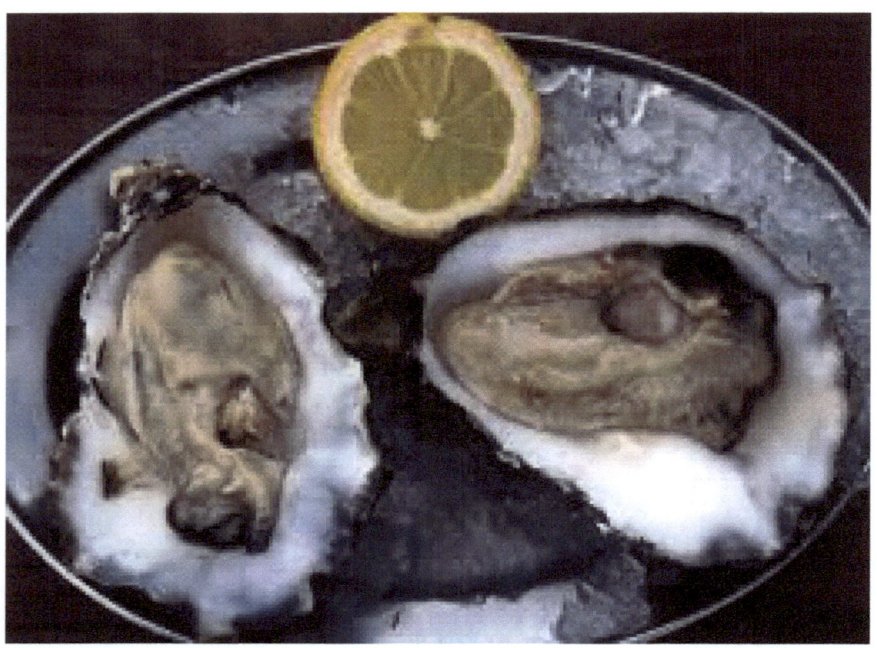

Fruits

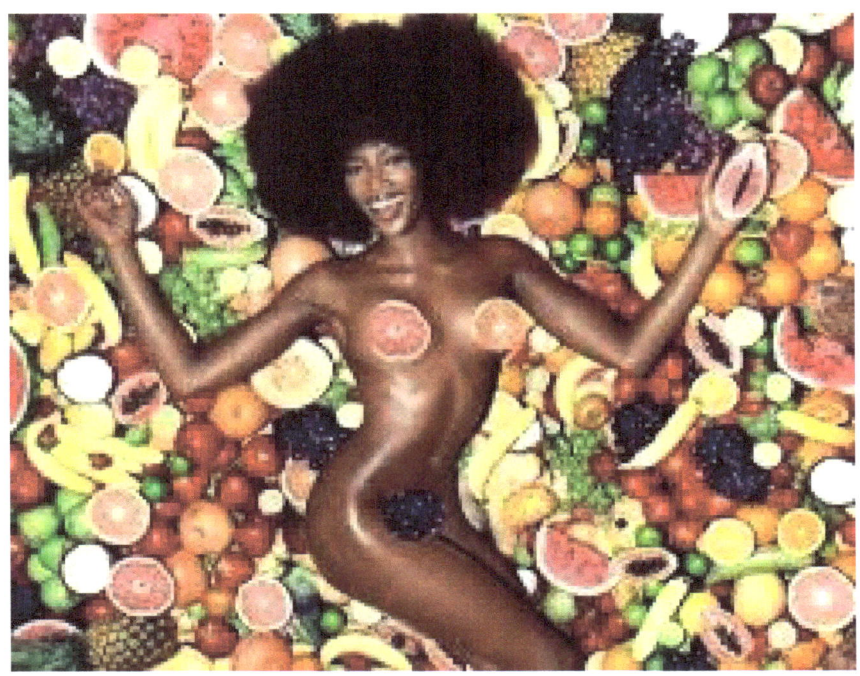

Fruits are undoubtedly a healthy way to spark arousal for love. These include, apricots, cherries, coconut, dates, figs, grapes, oranges, lemons, limes, mangoes, papayas, peaches, kiwi, pears, plums and pomegranate. In particular, the forbidden fruit of apples, and the potassium rich bananas, can give energy when it is most required. Another fruit that is known for boosting your sex drive is avocado, which is rich in vitamin E.

Some berries are very beneficial, such as blueberries which are high in vitamin B and encourage healthy sexual function, raspberries which enhance sexual arousal, and of course the most symbolic fruit of love, strawberries, especially with chocolate! The seeds of these latter berries are rich in zinc, which boosts testosterone in men and helps women get in the mood for love.

Vegetables

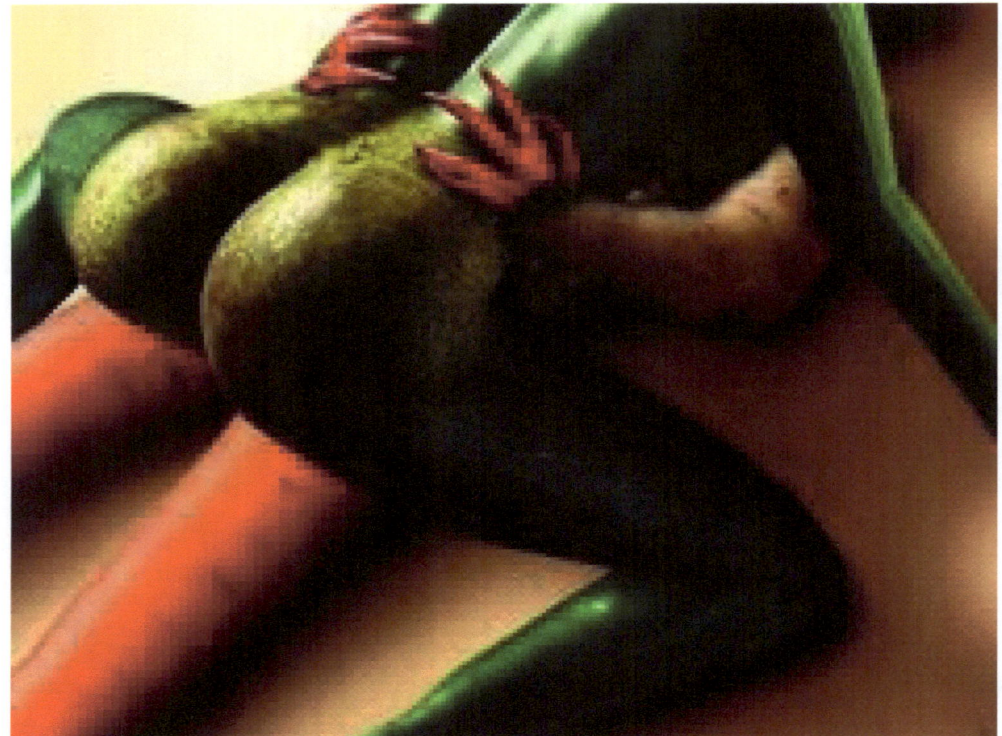

Vegetables that a well known for their aphrodisiac properties include, asparagus, spinach, carrots, celery, bean sprouts, corn, chillies, artichokes, cucumbers, broccoli, Swiss chard, leafy greens, onions, garlic, ginger, aubergine (eggplant), courgettes and fresh salads. Pumpkin seeds are very good for sex because they are high in zinc. Too many potatoes are not recommended, especially fried.

Nuts

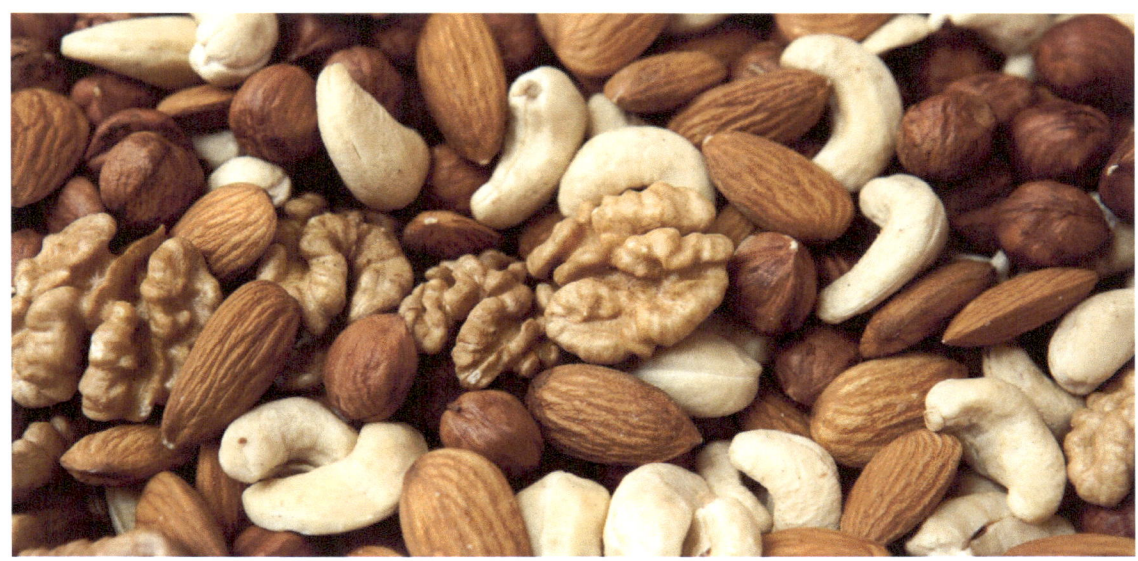

Nuts can hugely boost your sex drive because nuts like almonds are bursting with essential fatty acids that help maintain a healthy balance of sex hormones. Brazil nuts are great for men as they are a major source of selenium, a vitamin that helps keep sperm cells healthy. Others include cashews, walnuts and peanuts.

Meats and Fish

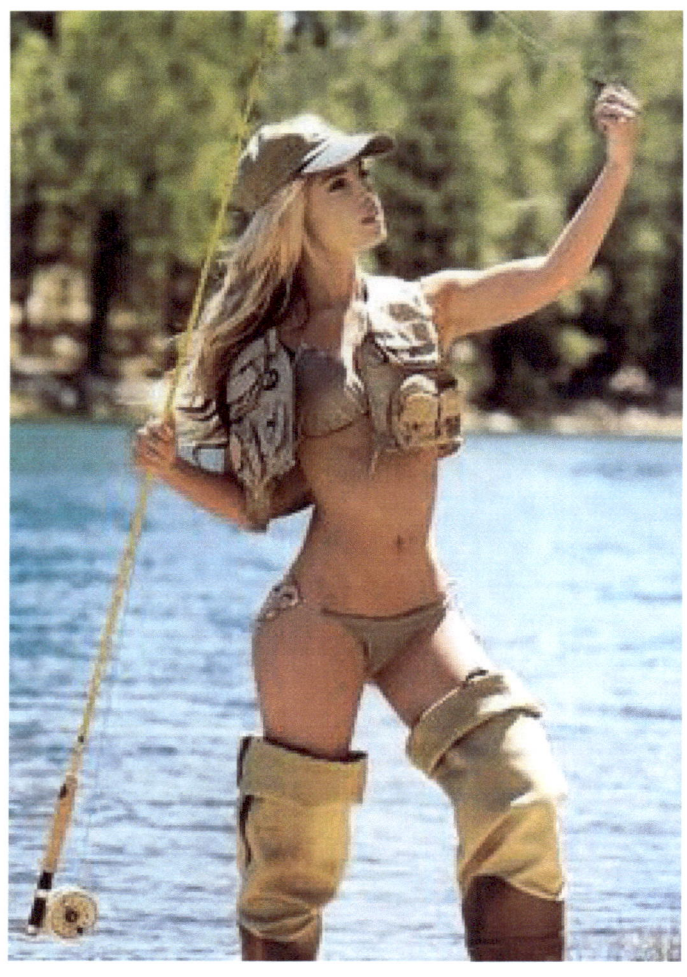

Lean red meat, liver, egg yolks, fat-less chicken and turkey, sushi, and oily fish which is high in omega 3, can all aid your love making. In particular, oysters are well known for their aphrodisiac properties because they are the richest food source of zinc.

Chocolate

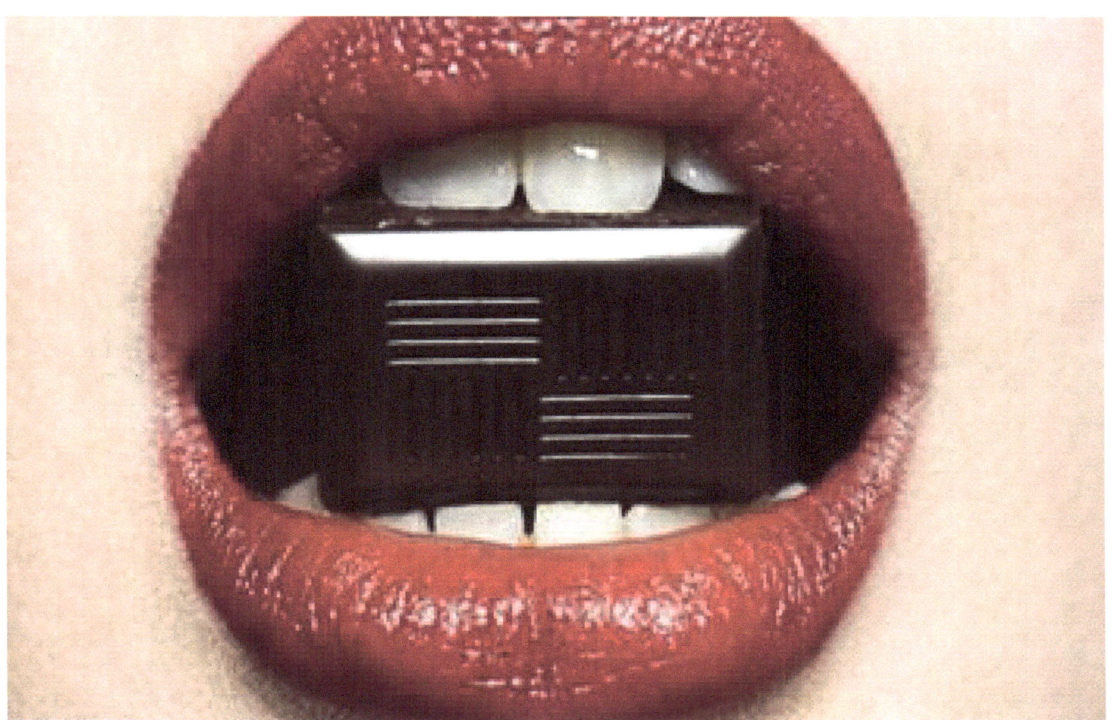

When it comes to making love, chocolate can't be ignored. It is often referred to as a "love drug." Use it as a sauce or as sweets or even in cakes, it will, certainly melt hearts and bring the two of you closer. Chocolate contains phenylalanine, an amino acid that increases the body's endorphins and natural antidepressants. It can also increase blood flow to all the right places, increasing sexual desire. Go for at least 70% cocoa solids and dark chocolate.

If you want to be erotically bold and experimental, try using a chocolate sauce or whipped cream to paint your lover, and then lick away!

Drinks

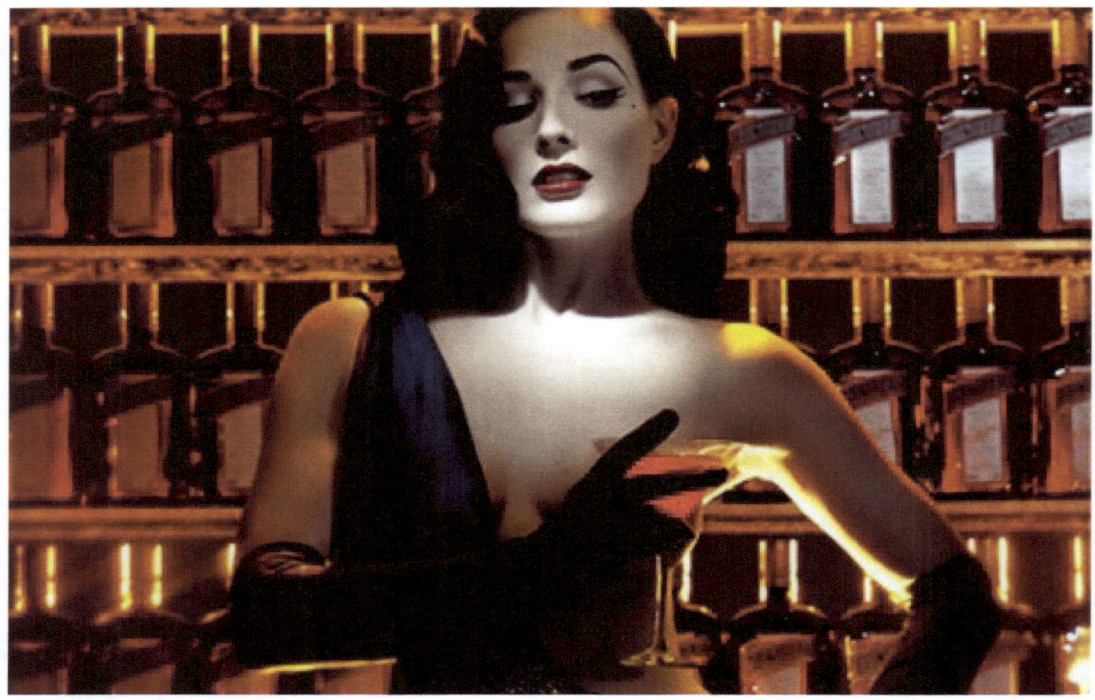

A night of passion can always be intensified with the addition of a favourite wine. What better way than sipping luscious red wine to give your time together a relaxed mood. Naturally, if you can get hold of vintage brands like Sassella, Brunellos and a nice French Chateau, it is adds to the occasion. Champagne is also known for its sexual properties. Wines are better than spirits or beer, because too much alcohol can affect your sexual performance too.

If wine is not your thing, you also have large choice of fresh fruit drinks, fruit smoothies and soft drinks like Slice (aamsutra), Appletiser, Sholer, Carpe Diem as alternatives.

Not all foods are great for enhancing your sex life. For example, fried, oily, fatty food and rich cream sauces can leave you feeling more sluggish than sexy. Interestingly, foods that are excessive sugar, salt, saturated fat and highly processed foods are related to frigidity, difficulty reaching orgasm and slowing down sex drive dramatically.

So, it's best to eat more of the wholesome sexy foods to give your love life a well deserved boost!

STARTER: Steamy asparasex

Ingredients

1 bunch asparagus

3 tbsp lemon juice

2 tbsp olive oil (not extra virgin)

Pinch of cayenne pepper

Pinch of white pepper

1 tsp capers, chopped

100 g fresh white crabmeat

Salt

Remove the woody ends from the asparagus

Bring a pan of water to the boil, add the asparagus, and simmer for 3 minutes. Drain and refresh under cold water.

Make the vinaigrette by whisking together the lemon juice and olive oil until emulsified. Add the cayenne pepper, white pepper, and a little salt. Stir in the capers and crabmeat. Taste and add more seasoning if required.

To serve, divide the asparagus spears between two plates and spoon half the dressing over each, making sure you distribute the crabmeat evenly.

MAIN: Drunken Figs

Ingredients

6 ripe figs

2 tbsp honey

2 tbsp of brandy

4 tbsp fat Greek

Zest of 1 orange

Light grating of nutmeg

Preheat the oven to 180°C/Gas 4.

Cut the figs in half lengthwise and arrange them in a shallow baking dish, close together. Attempt to evenly distribute the honey over them, followed by your booze of choice.

Cover and bake in the oven for approximately 20 minutes, or until softened.

Mix together the yogurt and orange zest and serve with the figs.

DRINK: The Mexican Boozer

Ingredients

125ml of cold water

125g dark chocolate, broken into small pieces

1 tbsp fine caster sugar

1/2 tsp vanilla extract

Pinch of chili powder

Pinch of salt

2 shots dark rum

2 cinnamon sticks

Place all the ingredients except the cinnamon sticks and rum in a pan and place over a medium heat, stirring constantly. The chocolate is ready when everything is dissolved and it is hot but not boiling.

Pour the rum into mugs, followed by the chocolate mixture. To serve, add a cinnamon stick to each mug; this can be used every now and then to stir up any chocolate which has dared to settle on the bottom.

Main: Steamy Fish

Ingredients

Ice

2 spring onions green parts only, cut into thin strips

1 red chili, cut into thin strips

2 x 160g fillets of sea bass

2.5cm piece of ginger, peeled and cut into very thin matchsticks

1 tbsp groundnut oil

2 tsp sesame oil

1.5 tbsp soy sauce

A few small sprigs fresh coriander

Salt

Fill a bowl with water and add a good handful or two of ice.

Throw the spring onions and chili strips into it and in 15 minutes or so they will all have curled up. This will make the finished dish look great. Drain and dry on a paper towels.

Put the fish fillets on a plate and scatter with the ginger pieces. Pour over the soy sauce and let sit for 15 minutes.

Set a steamer basket over a pan of simmering water and place the fish fillets inside, leaving the ginger strips on the fish. Sprinkle over a pinch of salt. Steam for 8 minutes, then turn off the heat while you prepare the oil.

Heat the groundnut and sesame oils in a pan and add the chili strips; cook for about a minute. Place the fish fillets on a plate in the middle of the table and scatter over the spring onions. Pour the chili oil over the fish and you're done.

Artichoke, Lemon & Parmesan Pasta

Ingredients

150g spaghetti

100g marinated (drained and sliced) artichoke hearts

1 lemon (juiced and zested)

25g finely grated Parmesan

shredded basil and some olive oil.

Mix the artichoke, Parmesan, basil and lemon with a tablespoon of olive oil, season well with herbs (if desired) and toss them together with the (boiled) spaghetti. Serves two.

Chocolate Mousse With Chili

Ingredients

2 eggs (whites and yolk separated)

1 shot of espresso

1 tbsp powdered sugar

a pinch of powdered chili

2 tbsp unsalted butter

100gdark chocolate and whipped cream.

Melt the chocolate in an oven-safe bowl resting over a saucepan of simmering water, add the espresso and mix until smooth. Turn off the heat and mix in the butter, powdered chilli and egg yolks. Leave to cool. In a separate bowl, beat the egg whites and a pinch of salt until it foams, and add in the sugar while continuing to beat for a few more minutes.

Mix this into the bowl of chocolate (a little at a time), folding the egg whites into the chocolate gently until you have a light and creamy mousse. Pour into a serving bowl and let it rest in the fridge for 3-4 hours. Enjoy it with whipped cream.

Persephone

Ingredients

Lime juice

lavender sugar (mixture of dried ground lavender and fine sugar)

100ml pomegranate juice

100 ml mango elixir (mango concentrate and distilled water)

100ml syrup (equal parts sugar and water)

soda water

Dip the mouth of your glass into the lime juice. Add the pomegranate juice, followed by the mango elixir, syrup and finish with soda water and ice. Add a splash of your favourite spirit if you want some help dropping your inhibition.

Stove-top Method

This method is ideal for fresh herbs or if you are in a hurry.

1. Measure 1 cup honey per 2 tablespoon of chopped fresh herb (or 1 tbs dried)

2. Pour your honey into a double boiler. (If you don't have a double boiler you can easily create one by placing the ring part of the lid of a mason jar in a large pan. Fill with water until the ring is covered. Then, balance a smaller pot on top of the ring. The goal is to have the bottom of that smaller pot submerged in water, but not touching the very hot bottom of the pot containing the water).

3. Put your burner to medium/low heat. Once your honey is warm, add herbs and stir to distribute.

4. Let your honey sit for 1-6 hours. The longer it sits, the stronger it will be.

If you are leaving your honey for several hours, make sure to keep the smaller pot sitting in water. Add more water to your larger pot from time-to-time and don't forget to stir! You want your honey to stay warm enough that you could comfortably put it on your skin.

5. When it tastes scrumptious, you are done. (Word of Warning: because the honey will be very warm, all the flavors won't immediately jump out at you. Once it cools the taste will manifest 3-fold. If it's still not strong enough for your tastes, try adding a fresh batch of herbs and reheating).

6. Strain your herb from the honey while it is still hot (once it cools down you ain't ever gettin those herbs out). Use a piece of cheesecloth or fine mesh strainer and strain over a large bowl or directly into jars.

Sun Method

This method is lovely for any dried or delicate herbs

Get a clean, DRY jar. (If the jar isn't dry you risk inviting mold into your honey).

2. Put your herbs in the jar first and then pour honey over them. (It gets a lot messier the other way around)

3. Place your jar in a sunny window for one to two weeks…. or longer! If you're feeling ambitious, turn the jar over each day to re-distribute the herbs.

4. I would recommending heating the honey just slightly in order to strain the herbs.

Elixirs

Elixirs are basically a fancy name for an alcohol and honey infusion. There are several different ways to make an elixir and, as for combinations, the sky is the limit

Method 1: Separate but Equal

1. Make your infused honey (see process above)

2. Combine different tinctures (or just use a simple) to get the alcohol base.

3. Mix together your honey and tincture formula until it tastes just right. Fini!

Not sure how to make a tincture? Here is the fabulously easy folk method way of making alcohol extracts

1. Purchase the highest quality alcohol you can find (lots of people like using 190 proof vodka. If you prefer a milder extraction, try brandy or whiskey. If you plan on making a lot of tinctures I highly recommended buying pharmaceutical grade organic alcohol online. Alchemical solutions is a wonderful company!

2. If you are using fresh herbs chop finely (or grind) and put into a jar. Fill the jar 2/3-3/4 full with herbs (if using roots fill ¼-1/2 full)

3. Pour enough alcohol into the jar to cover the herbs. Cap, label and store in a dark place for at least 6 weeks. Visit your tincture from time to time to give it a little shake and a good snuggle.

3. If you are using dry herb fill you jar only ½ to ¾ with herb (only ¼ to 1/3 if its roots). Pour alcohol over the herbs to fill the jar (You want about a 1:4 ratio of herb to liquid. If you want to get real fancy, have 60% of that liquid be alcohol and the remaining 40% water. Since dry herb lacks water, it will expand and take up some of that extra fluid.)

Method 2: All Together Now

1. Fill a jar with your herb material. It doesn't have to be completely packed, but it should be full enough that there isn't much airspace (fresh or dry is fine).

2. Pour enough honey in to completely coat the herb. (Usually the ratio is about 1:3 volume for fresh herbs. So for a pint of lemonbalm you might use 1/3 pint of honey)

3. Once the herb is coated, pour your alcohol in to fill the remainder of the jar.

4. Cap your mixture and put in a cool dark place for 3-6 weeks. (You can use plastic wrap underneath the jar lid to make sure no extra air is sitting at the top and to avoid that metallic taste)

5. Strain, or don't strain. It's all up to you. If you do decide to strain and want to heat the honey, just be aware that some of the alcohol content will evaporate off.

Damiana Spice Tea

1 part damiana leaf

1 part rose petals

1/2 part spearmint leaf

¼ each: cinnamon chips, licorice root, ginger root, whole cloves

Sweet Heart Blend

1 part rose petals

1 part tulsi

½ part rose hips

½ part hawthorn berries

¼ each: ginger root, cinnamon & vanilla bean

pinch cardamom

Divine Love Honey Spice of Life Honey

1 part cinnamon 1 part cinnamon

1 part star anise 1 part ginger

1 part coriander ½ cardamom pods (if powder try ¼ ratio)

½ orange peel ¼ cayenne

¼ ginger

¼ vanilla bean

Damiana Chocolate Love Liqueur

1 ounce damiana leaves (dried)

2 cups vodka or brandy

1 ½ cups spring-water

1 cup honey

vanilla extract

rose water

chocolate syrup

almond extract

1. Soak the damiana leaves in the vodka or brandy for 5 days. Strain. Reserve the liquid in a bottle

2. Soak the alcohol-drenched leaves in the spring-water for 3 days. Stain and reserve the liquid

3. Over low heat, gently warm the water extract and dissolve honey in it. Remove the pan from the heat, then add the alcohol extract and stir well. Pour into a clean bottle and add a dash of vanilla and a touch of rose water for flavor. Let it mellow for 1 month or longer; it gets smoother with age

4. To each cup of damiana liqueur, add ½ cup of chocolate syrup, 2 or 3 drops of almond extract, and a touch more of rose water

Rose Petal Elixir

1 pint Mason jar

Fresh wild or domestic rose petals to fill your jar (make sure they have not been

A little less than 1 pint of good quality brandy (or vodka. if using higher proof booze dilute with 50% water)

1/3 pint of raw honey

1. Fill your jar with fresh rose petals. They don't have to be packed down, but they should fill the jar so that there isn't a lot of empty space.

2. If you don't have enough rose petals to fill the jar, you could add some bee balm petals, chopped fresh ginger, zest of orange, lime, or lemon, etc.

3. Next, add honey to coat the rose petals and fill about 1/3 of the jar. Add brandy or other alcohol to the top of the jar. Place plastic wrap over the top and then screw on your metal lid. (if you don't your mixture might start tasting metallic. Alcohol and roses are particularly adept at taking on those flavors) Allow to sit in a cool, dark place for 3-6 weeks before using.

Well that's it for now, just a short insight into some of the sexiest foods on earth.